hCG Diet Secrets

How to Lose 30 Pounds In 30 Days

By: Patricia L. Steele

Patricia L. Steele

Exclusive Bonus Resource for Readers of Hcg Diet Secrets

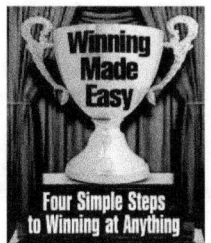 ✔ Discover the 4 Steps to Winning Everyday in Every Way in your life right now!

✔ Learn how you can make money consistently and effortlessly even in this economy.

✔ Get insider secrets to attracting and keeping your soul mate happy!

Visit http://goo.gl/sQZg9n to claim your above FREE exclusive bonus content.

TABLE OF CONTENTS

Patricia L. Steele

PUBLISHERS NOTES

Content in this publication is for reference purposes and is not intended to substitute for advice given by a physician, pharmacist, or other licensed health-care professional. You should not use this information as self-diagnosis or for treating a health problem or disease.

Contact your health-care provider immediately if you suspect that you have a medical problem. Information and statements regarding dietary supplements have not been evaluated by the Food and Drug Administration and are not intended to diagnose, treat, cure, or prevent any disease or health condition. The publisher Argon Media LLC and the author assumes no liability for inaccuracies or misstatements in this product.

Terms of Use

You are given a non-transferable, "personal use" license to this product. You cannot distribute it or share it with other individuals.

Also, there are no resale rights or private label rights granted when purchasing this document. In other words, it's for your own personal use only.

INTRODUCTION

With the vast majority of weight loss diet plans available today, there is a noticeable trend in limiting calorie intake and restricting certain foods. This includes high protein/low carb diets, like the Atkins diet. It also includes short-term fad diets, like the grapefruit diet or the cabbage soup diet.

The result of these fad diets often ends up slowing down your metabolic rate even further. The body goes into starvation mode as it perceives that food is being limited. This immediately sends a signal to the body to begin storing any food that is consumed as fat stores. This is a primitive response that stems back from our ancestors during times of food shortages.

For this reason, the pharmaceutical industry loves to promote 'miracle' weight loss pills, supplements and shakes. These things are advertised as making it easy to lose weight, but anyone who has tried them knows they simply don't work.

The reason they don't work is written right on the side of the package. Every one of those amazing miracle diet products has the same advice written somewhere on the label. They all say:

"Effective when used in conjunction with a calorie controlled diet and regular exercise"

That's wise advice. If you were to reduce your calorie intake and exercise more often, of course you'll start losing weight. This means the pills, supplements or shakes you think will help actually do nothing on their own.

It's also why all those fad diets don't work. The short term weight loss you might see on the bathroom scale might show that you've lost a few pounds, but you're not actually losing that wobbly body fat. Instead, you're more likely to be losing water and muscle tissue as your body looks for more efficient sources of fuel.

The moment you stop these diets, the weight immediately piles back on again. This is simply because you never lost any of the body fat stored around your body, but your body began to burn muscle tissue as a source of fuel. When you begin to lose muscle tone, you immediately look even more overweight than you really are. The fat deposits around your body become more pronounced, showing up as dimpled, wobbly, flabby flesh.

Far too many people believe that muscle weighs more than fat. They also believe that fat can be turned into muscle. Neither of these things are true. Fat cells will always be fat cells, and they can expand and shrink depending on how much energy they need to store. Muscle cells will always be muscle cells and even they can expand and contract.

And one pound of fat weighs exactly the same amount as one pound of muscle.

The difference is that muscle is far more dense than fat. Think about this: if you had 10 pounds of coins and 10 pounds of feathers, which will be bigger? They both weigh the same amount, but you need a lot more feathers to make up 10 pounds. The same is true with fat and muscle.

So, the key to real weight loss that stays off over the long term is to lose those fat deposits. This is the reason why so many people try crash diets and miracle diet pills and supplements and meal replacements. It's why they try fad diets that never seem to work.

However, there is an alternative. For more than 60 years, researchers have been aware of the effect of hCG treatments for fast, effective weight loss. While researchers know all about it, many medical doctors remained unaware of it. These doctors would ignore the comments from their patients that simply nothing works for them and recommend low calorie, low fat diets coupled with exercise for their patients to lose weight.

It's only in more recent years that Kevin Trudeau revived the interest in the hCG diet, simply because it works.

SUSPEND YOUR DOUBTS

There's a story about a woman named Jill who personifies suspending your doubts. When Jill was growing up she longed to be healthy and in shape. Instead she found herself where many other teens find themselves today -- on the other end of being popular, well liked and fitting in.

One day, she grew weary of all the taunts and negative names she had assailed her way. She wanted things to be different but she didn't know how to make that happen. She longed for riding horses, and despite the amount of physical activity that required, she just didn't have the fitness, stamina or self-esteem to pull it off.

For years she medicated her pain with food. She longed to be loved, liked and admired but somebody, but whenever you don't love yourself, it's hard for anybody else to find something of value inside of you.

After her teenage years, Jill kept with her desire to be healthy, fit and in control of her body. As things progressed, she finally found what worked.

It was not at the end of some doctor's surgery center, but she decided to make health and fitness her lifelong pursuit.

You probably know Jill as the tough as nails personal trainer on the hit television show, "The Biggest Loser". And you guessed it, Jill is Jillian Michael. Author, Fitness Star, Model, Healthy Lifestyle Advocate and Biggest Loser Personal Trainer.

She has come a long way from being taunted by unhealthy peers, and medicating her pain with food.

If Jillian Michaels did it, so can you.

Live true to your dream...

Napoleon Hill said, "All achievement and earthly riches have their beginnings in an idea or dream."

---Napoleon Hill

The story of Jillian emphasizes the magical power of your mind to suspend doubt and get into action. Did it take unpacking a lot of negative information she had heard about herself? Yes in-deed. Anything worth-while, requires effort!

Jillian is no different than you are. You've probably had many doubts about 'keeping the weight off.' No doubt, you've tried 'everything' but nothing seems to work.

Suspend your doubts. Start over. Double your efforts. Sometimes it is when we are about to give up the fight that a break through comes in for us.

You've got everything to gain. Look at Jillian. She did it. So can you. She was willing to unlearn much of what she thought, felt and knew was in her reality. When she weighed herself, the scales did not lie. She was overweight. She had no energy. She ate emotionally. She consumed carbs and did not work them off.

This is the key to lifelong body management. Love yourself enough to learn the truth. Then once you've found your truth, work with it. Don't quit. Don't give up because the best of you is yet to come.

Patricia L. Steele

SUSPEND your doubts! Procrastinate your doubts. Plan to do it tomorrow.

WHAT IS THE HCG DIET?

hCG is the acronym for Human Chorionic Gonadotropin, which is a naturally occurring human hormone that is usually found within pregnant women. The hormone is produced shortly after conception by the embryo. When a home pregnancy test kit is used, the strip actually tests for the presence of hCG in order to give a positive result. As the pregnancy progresses, the placenta begins to produce the hormone.

Back in the early 1950s, Dr. A. T. W. Simeons published a report about his studies on obesity. His research led to him creating the diet that came to be known as the hCG diet.

Throughout his research, he administered small doses of hCG to his patients. During their treatments, patients were limited to a very low-calorie diet, with the hCG treatments acting as supplements. As the study progressed, he noticed that his patients were losing a lot of weight very rapidly without having to exercise at all. Their bodies began to reshape naturally, with contours appearing as the amount of body fat decreased.

Another major finding within his studies was that the metabolic rate within his patients began to increase. Many overweight and obese patients have sluggish metabolisms at best, which usually means that it's more difficult for these people to burn off any excess calories they consume.

The result of being on the hCG diet for the vast majority of patients was that they lost weight rapidly, many of them losing between 1 and 3 pounds per day. Fat deposits began to shrink, leaving behind a more sculpted figure. Patients reported feeling immediately more energetic.

Once the diet was completed, patients found that their stomachs had shrunk down to normal size. This allowed them to resume eating a healthy diet with normal portion sizes, which also allowed them to keep the weight off over the long term.

HEALTH BENEFITS OF LOSING WEIGHT

The negative effects of being overweight or obese have been documented extremely well in the media over recent years. People who struggle with long term obesity face a greatly increased risk of developing some serious health conditions that may otherwise have been avoided. These include:

- Type 2 Diabetes

- Heart disease and atherosclerosis

- Stroke

- High blood pressure

- High cholesterol levels

- Blood circulation problems

- Asthma-related inflammation

- Joint inflammation and osteoarthritis

- Bowel cancer

- Infertility

- Pre-menstrual cramping and pain

- Constipation

- Depression

- Sleep apnea

\-   And many more besides!

By losing weight, the risk of developing these health conditions is greatly reduced.

Improving your overall health is a great motivation for wanting to lose weight. But there are some other benefits to losing weight that people don't tend to focus on.

When you start losing weight, you should notice that your self-esteem and self-confidence begin to improve. This helps you look and feel much better about yourself, but it also goes a little deeper than that.

You see, as you get your metabolism functioning properly again, you'll notice that your skin appears healthier and your hair will develop a natural sheen. If you suffer with acne problems, these will start to clear up. These simple things can make you appear radiant, almost as though you're glowing with happiness.

Increasing your metabolic rate also means you'll have more energy throughout the day. As your energy levels increase, you'll suddenly find that you wake up feeling refreshed and alive.

What's more, you'll be doing more with your day, which releases endorphins. These are your body's natural 'feel good' chemicals that help you reduce stress, reduce depression and make you feel naturally happy.

Many overweight and obese women also struggle with fertility problems. Simply by losing weight using a healthy plan, you reduce your risk of infertility enormously. There's also the benefit of reducing the severity of pre-menstrual cramping and avoiding those unpredictable mood swings.

Of course, there is one other big benefit to losing weight naturally and healthily, and that's the financial benefit. Research published in the Unites States in 2010 showed that people with a Body Mass Index (BMI) higher than 30 made up 17% of the entire $168 billion US medical expenditure for 2009. This is the same research that showed an extra $3,800 each year was spent on morbidly obese patients as compared to patients within a normal weight range.

Then there's the research from the United States that showed obese people earn 26% less than people within a normal weight range. This is most likely due to more sick days taken and lower productivity levels, which led to a reduced likelihood of being promoted to better paying jobs.

So, with so many physical, emotional and financial benefits to losing weight, it's time to do something positive about it. It's time to start the hCG diet and get that extra weight off once and for all.

Patricia L. Steele

POTENTIAL hCG SIDE EFFECTS

As hCG is a naturally occurring hormone produced by the human body, there are no reported toxic effects.

However, as with any form of medication, there is always going to be a potential risk for side effects that may occur. Some of these are incredibly positive side effects. Yet, some people may experience some adverse side effects.

Positive side effects that can occur with the hCG diet include:

-        Reduced risk of breast cancer: studies conducted at the University of Pennsylvania have shown that hCG can actively reduce growth within breast tumors. It also stimulated that production of genes and cells that cause breast cancer cysts to grow.

-        Stabilized Blood Sugar Levels: in people experiencing unstable blood sugar levels, the effects of being on the hCG diet resulted in blood sugar level improvements. This reduces the risk of developing Type 2 Diabetes in pre-diabetic women.

-        Increased Metabolic Rate: your metabolic rate is the rate at which your metabolism helps to burn fat. Many overweight people have a very sluggish metabolic rate, which makes losing weight more difficult. Reports from many people show that after being on the hCG diet their metabolic rate had improved, which accelerated their weight loss efforts.

-        Improved Self Confidence: the rapid weight loss results provided by the hCG diet have actively improved the self-confidence and self-esteem for those women using it. This results in a far more positive body image overall, which also resulted in a reported reduction in depression symptoms.

Negative side effects that may occur while on the hCG diet include:

-        Injection Site Soreness: some people do report a level of discomfort or sensitivity around the injection site for a short time. This may include swelling or irritation around the area where the injection was given.

-        Breast Tenderness: there are some reports of breast tenderness or swelling in some women on the hCG diet.

-        Headache: some women report a persistent headache while taking hCG. This is a common complaint for many people as your body adjusts to the reduced calorie intake and the fluctuations in your blood sugar levels. The moment your body adjusts to burning fat stores as an energy source instead of carbohydrates, the headaches will disappear.

-        Diarrhea: There have been a few reports of women experiencing diarrhea while on the hCG diet. If this symptom persists longer than a couple of days, it's important to seek medical advice.

Unfortunately, there are also a very small number of women who may develop more serious side effects while on the hCG diet. While these more severe side effects are not common, they include:

-        Swelling of the face, lips, tongue or throat

-        Pelvic pain, lower abdominal pain and swelling

-        Shortness of breath

Patricia L. Steele

As with any change in your diet, it's very important to seek medical advice. Explain to your doctor exactly what's involved in the hCG diet and what you intend to do. Always gain medical clearance before you begin this diet.

STARTING THE HCG DIET

There are three phases to the hCG diet that last for six weeks that you need to work through in order to see real results. Phase One includes loading days. Phase Two is the actual dieting phase, and Phase Three is when you maintain your diet for another three days without the hCG supplements.

Let's walk through each phase to be absolutely sure you get all the steps correct.

Before You Begin...

Before you start taking your hCG supplements, it's important to prepare your body for a change in diet. The original creator of the hCG diet intended for this to be a low calorie diet back in 1954. However, when the diet was revived again in 2007, Kevin Trudeau noticed that many of the foods we eat today are changed.

Fresh foods are now pumped full of pesticides and herbicides, along with chemically-created fertilizers and growth stimulants. Other food types are pumped full of antibiotics and hormones, among other things. Pre-packaged foods are filled with preservatives, artificial coloring and flavoring, and chemical additives.

For this reason, it might be a wise idea to consider using good quality supplements to ensure you're getting the right nutrients, vitamins and minerals and to help increase the effects of your diet.

You should also consider switching coffee, tea or soda with water. If you really can't stand to drink plain water throughout your day, find an organic green tea you prefer instead. Green tea is extremely good for you and provides plenty of health benefits all on its own.

An Important Note about Menstruation

Patricia L. Steele

It is very important that you stop taking all your hCG injections during menstruation, but you should still stick firmly to the diet meal plans and portion sizes through this time.

When your period has ended you will feel abnormally hungry. Don't be tempted to break your diet here. Instead, you can resume taking your injections again. You should find that the hunger pangs stop within a couple of hours after taking your hCG injection.

hCG Diet Food Guidelines

While you're on the hCG diet, it's important to choose the right foods to eat. The meal plans available aren't set in stone, so it's fine to eat a satisfying meal that fits within the diet guidelines set out.

The key to getting this right is to remember that some foods are okay and others should be completely avoided.

Don't Eat These Foods

-        Sugar: sweet, sugary foods need to be avoided. If you have a sweet tooth, look for sugar-free options to sooth those cravings.

-        Fats: if you're preparing meat for your meal, always be sure to remove all visible fat before you cook it. This will result in leaner meat, but it's impossible to remove it all so this will be fine.

-        Oils: don't use any oils in your cooking and never fry your food while you're on the hCG diet. Wherever possible, grill your food or stir-fry it lightly. Kevin Trudeau suggests that coconut oil is fine.

-        Carbohydrates: your body really does need some carbohydrates in order to survive, but you should remove major sources of these where you can. This includes potatoes, bread and pasta.

-        Processed or Pre-packaged Foods: wherever possible, try to avoid processed or pre-packaged foods. It's very easy to make your own healthy meals, so avoid anything that contains artificial additives and preservatives. These also tend to contain high amounts of sodium and sugar.

Eat These Foods For hCG Success

There are some foods that are ideal when added to your daily meal plans. These include:

-        Chicken: chicken is an ideal meat source while you're on the hCG diet. Just be sure you grill it and not fry it.

-        Fish and Seafood: fish and seafood are excellent sources of Omega 3 Fatty Acids, which are healthy essential acids your body needs to function optimally.

-        Lean beef or veal: if you do choose to eat beef or veal, always be sure to remove all visible fat before you cook it.

-        Leafy greens: lettuce and spinach are always find to add to salads, meal recipes and side dishes at any time.

-        Legumes: peas, beans and lentils are an excellent choice for any meal plan.

-        Fruit: grapes, strawberries, bananas, apples, oranges and most other fruits will make excellent healthy snacks throughout your day.

-        Vegetables: Most vegetables are absolutely fine to add to your daily meal plans.

STEP BY STEP hCG DIET

There are three phases to the hCG diet that need to be followed as closely as possible. This will help to ensure you get the best weight loss results.

Phase One

Phase One is all about loading. For two entire days, you're encouraged to eat as much as you want until you're full. This sounds like an absolute dream for anyone about to start a diet, but there is a catch.

You see, the whole point of loading is to help your body make the transition from burning carbs over to burning your fat reserves instead. You also want to ensure that you don't end up suffering with headaches when you enter Phase Two.

For this reason, there is a list of recommended foods you should try to include in your Phase One loading days. You also need to remember the list of fatty, sugary or oily foods to avoid while you're on this diet, so you can't just eat anything you feel like. You do still have to stick to the recommended foods list.

For the first two days, go ahead and eat as much as you like of the following:

Meat:

-        Chicken

-        Lean turkey

-        Very lean beef

-        Tuna

- Mackerel

- Herring

- Trout

- Sardines

- Salmon

- Anchovies

- Prawns or shrimp

- Crab meat

Dairy:

- Cheese

- Cottage cheese

- Cream

- Whole eggs

- Milk

- Low fat Yogurt

Nuts and Seeds:

- Almonds

- Brazil Nuts

- Cashews

- Hazelnuts

- Macadamia nuts

- Peanuts

- Walnuts

- Flax seeds

- Pumpkin seeds

- Sunflower seeds

Fruit:

- Avocados

- Olives

- Any citrus fruit

- Any stone fruit

- Any other fruit

Vegetables:

Patricia L. Steele

-        Any vegetables

Remember, during the first two loading days you're allowed to eat as much as you like of any of the foods mentioned above. You're not restricted, so eat whenever you're hungry and eat until you're full.

Phase Two

During Phase Two, you begin taking your hCG supplements and you start with the eating plan laid out by Dr. Simeons and refined by Kevin Trudeau.

Phase Two can last anywhere from 26 to 40 days, depending on how much weight you want to lose and how long you want to remain on the diet.

Always remember that if a particular food is listed that you don't like or that you have a reaction to, don't eat it. Only include foods that agree with you.

The list of foods and the exact portion sizes are important during this phase. You can find an exact listing of these within Dr Simeons' 'Pounds and Inches' book.

The recommended foods include:

Vegetables: all vegetables are fine to include in your daily meal plan. Two cups is the approximate serving size before the vegetables are cooked. Just be sure you don't mix your vegetables, but ensure that you get two full servings per day.

Fruit: you do need to include two servings of fruit each day. Where possible, avoid eating the same type of fruit two days in a row.

Meat: measuring and weighing your portion sizes is important throughout the hCG diet. You should stick to servings that are no more than 3.5 ounces or 100 grams, so remove any visible fat from meat before you weigh and cook it.

Eggs: Eggs are allowed, but never two days in a row and never fried. Always prepare your eggs so they're poached, boiled or scrambled.

Bread: Limit your bread servings to two per day. Dr. Simeons recommends Melba toast or Grissini bread wherever possible.

Liquids: you're allowed to drink as much water as you want throughout the day. If you feel hungry, drink a glass of water as this will help to reduce hunger pangs. Organic green tea is also fine. You're only allowed one tablespoon of milk per day, so if you must drink coffee you will need to limit the amount of milk you use.

Phase Three

During Phase Three you stop taking your hCG supplements, but you continue eating the exact same food plan as in Phase Two. This phase lasts for three days and is designed to allow you to rid your body of the hCG.

If you've lost as much weight as you hoped to lose throughout Phase Two, this becomes your maintenance phase. Hopefully during your time on the diet you would have learned some healthier food habits and some healthier recipes that you can keep in your regular meal plans.

Keep the same meal plan and calorie count as you used throughout all of Phase Two for the entire three days. This is important!

After Your Diet

After the three days of Phase Three, you are encouraged to increase your calorie count a little. The extremely low calorie intake throughout the diet is designed to help you lose weight. Increasing your calories slightly after this time will maintain your new weight.

Always keep in mind that any foods included in the hCG diet are always fine to eat during your maintenance phase. You can increase your meat portion sizes a little and you can start to include a few more carbohydrates, such as potatoes, pasta and bread.

Don't make the mistake of thinking you can go back to eating anything you want. Heading straight back to fried foods or junk food or sugary treats will only result in you putting all that weight back on again. After all the hard work you've done, learn some ways to find healthier treats, snacks and desserts and you won't undo all your efforts.

Increasing Your Success Rate

When you're on any kind of weight loss diet, it can be difficult to stay motivated. Sometimes the results aren't always what you hope for. Other times the temptation to cheat a little and eat a snack gets too much.

Yet, there are some things you can do to increase your success rate and keep you motivated at the same time.

Create a Journal

It's difficult to know where you're going if you don't have an accurate starting point to work from. This is why creating a journal or a diary can be such a positive way to stay motivated and help you work through any other issues that might be challenging your resolve to stay on your diet.

Your journal needs to begin with your accurate measurements. This includes measurements for:

- Chest

- Upper arms

- Forearms

- Waist

- Hips

- Thighs

You also need to record your starting weight. If you can, include a 'before' photo of yourself wearing your underwear, or tight clothing that shows you exactly as you are before you begin. Don't worry about anyone else seeing this – it's just for you.

These entries give you a clear starting point, but they shouldn't be the only things you put into your journal entries.

It's important you write down why you're taking this journey and how you feel about yourself right at the beginning. Be honest about your reasons for wanting to begin the hCG diet and what you hope to achieve. After each day, write down your feelings about how you're proceeding with your diet plan.

When you're through the first week, jump onto the bathroom scale and weigh yourself. You should also take new body measurements to see if your body shape is beginning to change already. Record your new weight and measurements into your journal and see how far you've come already.

Waiting an entire week to check your results can be difficult for many people, but it's worth it in the end as it allows you to see the results of all your hard work. It also helps you to stay motivated for the week ahead.

Aside from this, waiting for that first week also allows you to look back through your journal and see any differences in your mood or energy levels from before you started your diet. You should be able to notice an immediate difference in energy levels, but many people also notice a difference in how positive or happy they feel within that week.

Maintain your journal throughout your entire diet plan. The differences you'll notice within yourself and your body will amaze you.

Know Your 'Why'

Wanting to lose weight so you look and feel better about yourself is a good thing. However, most overweight people don't know exactly 'why' they want to lose weight. Sure, they just don't want to be overweight any longer. They might want the freedom to buy clothing off the rack. They might simply want that sexy, lean body they had before having kids. They might also just want to improve their health and bring back that self-confidence again.

It makes absolutely no difference what the reason is. What is important is that you understand your reason 'why'. Write down exactly why you want to lose weight and don't hold back.

You may find that this brings up an emotional flood of things you might have suppressed for a long time, but it's important to get these things out.

Dig deep and write down everything being overweight makes you feel. Think carefully about why you want to lose weight and write down all the things you hope to achieve while you're on your diet.

After all, once you have a strong enough motivational force to drive you it becomes much easier to stay on track.

Accountability

When you start your diet, tell everyone around you. Ask them to support you in your efforts and make yourself accountable to them. You're far less likely to give into temptation when you – and you alone – are accountable for your final results.

Taking accountability for your own results makes it more difficult to find excuses to break your diet or cheat on your meal plan. It also inspires you to find additional ways to increase your success rate.

Learning from Mistakes

Never, ever scold or punish yourself for having a bad day with your diet. You're only human, so there's no need to believe you can do everything perfectly the first time.

If you ever have days where you break your meal plan or you cheat a little, don't fall into blame mode and give up on your diet.

Instead, write down what happened in your journal. Look for anything that might have sparked your tiny digression and write this down too. When you can spot what made you feel the way you did and what led you to having a bad day, it suddenly becomes much easier not to repeat the same mistake in future.

Rather than punishing yourself and becoming tempted to give up, learning from your mistakes and taking accountability for them makes you stronger. It makes it much easier for you to get back on the right track again and really get those results you're hoping for.

Ask for Support

It's not always easy to get friends and family to support you on "yet another diet", especially when they seem so very doubtful about your ability to stick with it. If you have people around you that you aren't comfortable asking for support, take heart.

There are so many hCG diet forums available, all filled with women who are going through exactly the same things you are. They understand and empathize with what you're doing and what you're trying to achieve.

Join a couple of these and actively ask for support. When you have people around you willing to offer helpful advice and words of encouragement, you'll find that success is much easier to achieve.

hCG Friendly Desserts

One of the biggest issues many women on the hCG diet face is that they crave a sweet treat for dessert after a main meal. Don't start thinking that you need to go completely without desserts the entire time – there is good news.

The key to making great desserts that satisfy that sweet tooth without ruining your diet is to choose carefully from the available food lists for Phase Two and Phase Three and then find recipes that match these.

Here are some suggestions that might help:

Mock Meringue Cookies

Ingredients:

3 egg whites

1 pinch of cream of tartar

1 pinch of salt

½ teaspoon of vanilla extract

Stevia to sweeten

Sprinkle of cinnamon

Method:

Preheat your oven to 250F (120C). In a medium sized bowl, beat the egg whites, cream of tartar, vanilla and salt until the mixture forms stiff peaks. Line a cookie sheet with grease-proof paper. Drop a teaspoon-full of mixture onto the sheet. Repeat until all the mixture is used up. Bake in the oven for 20 minutes. If the top isn't golden, you can place the cookies under the broiler or the griller for a few seconds. Be careful with this step and watch them carefully as they'll burn quickly.

Remove cookies from the oven and allow them to cool. Sprinkle with a little Stevia and a dash of cinnamon. Enjoy!

Baked Apple Delight

Ingredients:

1 apple

1 packet of Stevia

½ teaspoon cinnamon

Method:

Slice the apple into thin wedges and layer them in a microwave-safe bowl. Sprinkle the apple slices lightly with Stevia and cinnamon. Microwave the apples on high for 3 minutes.

Choc Drop Delight

Ingredients:

Patricia L. Steele

1 cup coconut oil

¾ cup cocoa powder

8 packets Stevia (1g packs)

Method:

Place coconut oil in a microwave safe bowl and heat on high for 15-20 seconds. This should be just enough to get it to turn to liquid. Add the cocoa powder and the Stevia and mix thoroughly until all ingredients are well combined.

Pour small amounts of the mixture into clean ice cube trays and place in the freezer for 30 minutes. Remove from the freezer and turn the choc drops out of the ice cube tray. Store any unused drops in the fridge until needed.

Strawberry Slushie

Ingredients:

8 frozen strawberries

Juice of 1 lemon

3 Stevia packs

¼ cup of water

Method:

Place the strawberries into a blender, along with the juice from 1 lemon and the Stevia packs. Pour about half of the water amount into the blender. Blend until all ingredients are well mixed. If more moisture is required to keep the blender working, pour a little more water in. Serve immediately.

Coffee Mint Choc Smoothie

Ingredients:

3/4 cup chilled strong coffee

Peppermint flavored Stevia

Chocolate flavored Stevia

¼ teaspoon cocoa powder

2 ice cubes

½ tablespoon skim milk

Method:

Place all ingredients into the blender and blend well until mixture is smooth. Serve immediately.

INCIDENTAL ACTIVITY

Accelerating your results is very possible, even though the hCG diet alone should give you the rapid weight loss effects that you want. The problem with losing so much weight so quickly is that your skin doesn't have the opportunity to shrink back into place as the fat layers beneath them start to recede.

This can result in sagging skin that appears flabby. You can remove some of this effect by adding just a little bit of incidental activity into your daily routine.

Incidental activity can be ideal for toning up those flabby areas so you can avoid the sagging effect of losing weight. As you tone up, you're helping to create a bit of muscle tone, which instantly helps to boost your metabolic rate at the same time.

An increased metabolic rate means you're burning fat more effectively, even when you're resting. As a result your weight loss efforts get even easier.

Research has shown conclusively that a bit of incidental activity done several times throughout your day can have the exact same effect as working up a sweat for an entire hour at the gym.

For example: if you do five minutes of physical activity several times a day, you're getting a full hour long work out by the end of that day.

So, you might park the car a little further away from the doors at the mall and walk for five minutes to get inside from the car. By the time you're done with your shopping, you get another five minute walk back across the car park. As you walk, remember to stand tall and hold in your abdominal muscles. This will help you to tone and flatten your stomach while you're walking without worrying about doing endless sit-ups or crunches. Walking taller can also help to tone up your calves, your thighs and your buttocks without too much effort at all.

While you're watching TV at night, you might grab a tin of soup out of the pantry and do five minutes of bicep curls for each arm during the commercial breaks. That's another 10 minutes worth of incidental activity squeezed into your day, and you'll be toning up your arms and shoulders while you sit.

As you drive, you might decide to do some isometric toning while you're stopped at each set of traffic lights. Isometric toning simply means you're working one set of muscles at a time. So, you might squeeze your butt cheeks together tightly and hold that for 10 seconds before releasing them. Repeat this a few times and you'll be toning up your buttocks while you drive.

When you're at home doing simple chores, use this as an opportunity to get some incidental activity done. Sweeping and mopping floors is boring, but if you turn on a favorite tune while you do these things, you can do a little jig while you work. That little bit of dancing around gets your heart pumping, which gets your endorphins flowing, which suddenly makes a boring task a bit more fun.

At the same time, you're adding to your daily level of incidental activity.

Adding just a little extra activity throughout each and every day is a sure way to help your body tone up as you lose weight. This is a quick and effective way to accelerate your weight loss efforts at the same time as toning up your body.

CONCLUSION

If you've already tried every diet and weight loss plan out there and not gotten the results you hoped for, it's understandable that you'll be naturally reluctant to try yet another one.

However, with such overwhelming research and evidence of how successful the hCG diet can be, it's worth the effort.

Always take the time to prepare your food list and your journal before you begin your diet. This helps you to get into the right frame of mind before you even begin. It also helps to improve your chances of success dramatically.

Be diligent about tracking your success in your journal and be accountable for the results you do or don't get.

When your diet is done and you've achieved the weight loss goals you hoped for, you'll be able to look back on your journey and know it was all worthwhile in the end.

We'd love to hear from you and share in your success. Please, if you will, send us an email and proclaim your success so that others may know and support you in phase 1, 2, 3 and beyond.

You can share with us and our readers at yourdietresults@gmail.com.

I look forward to hearing of your success!

Patricia =)

ABOUT THE AUTHOR

Patricia Steele is intimately familiar with a chronic diet failure. Much of the time and anguish she spent wondering why she was so different than others was simply unfounded. This lead her to research and document much of what she and others just like you have been experiencing for years.

Finally, here's something that works!

www.ingramcontent.com/pod-product-compliance
Lightning Source LLC
Chambersburg PA
CBHW061804280526
45787CB00003BA/1478